SPOTLIGHT ON OUR FUTURE

PANDEMICS: COVID-19 AND OUR WORLD

JILL KEPPELER

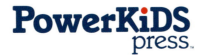

NEW YORK

Published in 2022 by The Rosen Publishing Group, Inc.
29 East 21st Street, New York, NY 10010

Copyright © 2022 by The Rosen Publishing Group, Inc.

All rights reserved. No part of this book may be reproduced in any form without permission in writing from the publisher, except by a reviewer.

First Edition

Editor: Greg Roza
Book Design: Michael Flynn

Photo Credits: Cover Drazen Zigic/Shutterstock.com; (series background) jessicahyde/Shutterstock.com; p. 4 Radoslav Zilinsky/Moment/Getty Images; p. 5 izusek/E+/Getty Images; p. 7 ePhotocorp/iStock/Getty Images; p. 8 DEA/G. DAGLI ORTI/De Agostini Picture Library/Getty Images; p. 9 Time Life Pictures/The LIFE Picture Collection/Getty Images; p. 11 Stock Montage/Archive Photos/Getty Images; p. 13 Anthony Kwan/Getty Images; p. 14 RichVintage/E+/Getty Images; p. 15 Frederic J. Brown/AFP/Getty Images; p. 17 Pier Marco Tacca/Getty Images; p. 18 Anadolu Agency/Getty Images; p. 19 Gary Hershorn/Getty Images; p. 21 MediaNews Group/Long Beach Press-Telegram/Getty Images; p. 22 The Washington Post/Getty Images; p. 23 Allen J. Schaben/Los Angeles Times/Getty Images; p. 25 damircudic/E+/Getty Images; p. 26 picture alliance/Getty Images; p. 27 Bloomberg/Getty Images; p. 29 Newsday LLC/Newsday/Getty Images.

Cataloging-in-Publication Data

Names: Keppeler, Jill.
Title: Pandemics: COVID-19 and our world / Jill Keppeler.
Description: New York : PowerKids Press, 2022. | Series: Spotlight on our future | Includes glossary and index.
Identifiers: ISBN 9781725332584 (pbk.) | ISBN 9781725332607 (library bound) | ISBN 9781725332591 (6 pack)
Subjects: LCSH: COVID-19 (Disease)--Juvenile literature. | Epidemics--Juvenile literature.
Classification: LCC RA644.C67 K47 2022 | DDC 614.5'92414--dc23

Manufactured in the United States of America

Some of the images in this book illustrate individuals who are models. The depictions do not imply actual situations or events.

CPSIA Compliance Information: Batch #CSPK22. For further information contact Rosen Publishing, New York, New York at 1-800-237-9932.

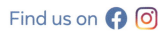

CONTENTS

A CHALLENGING TIME................................ 4
ABOUT VIRUSES 6
EPIDEMICS IN HISTORY 8
LEARNING FROM THE PAST 10
COVID-19 APPEARS 12
THE VIRUS SPREADS 14
WHAT HAPPENED IN ITALY 16
COMING TO AMERICA 18
COAST TO COAST.................................... 20
TAKING SIDES 22
THE ISSUE OF MASKS................................ 24
HOPE THROUGH SCIENCE............................. 26
LOOK FOR THE HELPERS 28
INTO THE FUTURE 30
GLOSSARY 31
INDEX 32
PRIMARY SOURCE LIST 32
WEBSITES... 32

CHAPTER ONE

A CHALLENGING TIME

Before 2020, most people probably didn't think much about the chances of an epidemic or pandemic occurring during their lifetime. However, on December 31, 2019, officials in Wuhan, China, first reported cases of COVID-19, an illness caused by a new virus. Within just a few days, more than 40 people had the illness. And soon, the first victim died from COVID-19.

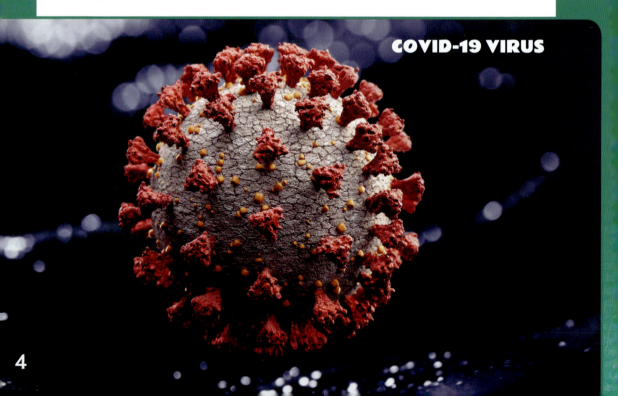

COVID-19 VIRUS

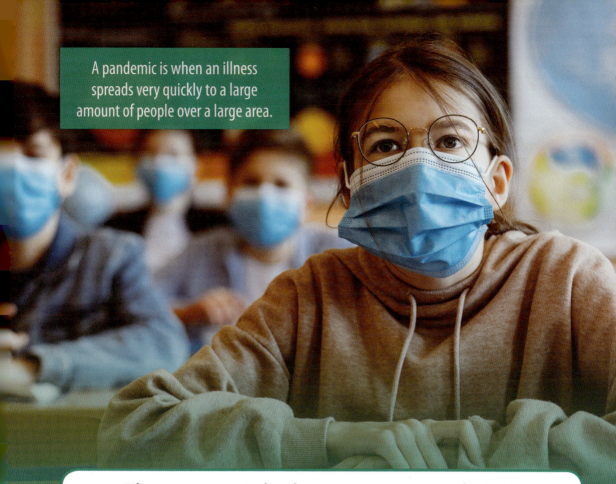

A pandemic is when an illness spreads very quickly to a large amount of people over a large area.

That was just the beginning. By early 2021, there had been more than 2 million deaths from COVID-19 around the world, with many millions of known cases of the sickness. Many people lost their jobs, kids missed school, and almost everyone's way of life had changed.

But there is hope. It's important to know how viruses work, what scientists have learned about them, and what you can do to help stop them from spreading.

CHAPTER TWO

ABOUT VIRUSES

Viruses are tiny **particles**, ones that can only be seen with powerful instruments. They can only grow, reproduce, and spread within living cells. COVID-19 is caused by a kind of virus called a coronavirus. A coronavirus also causes **influenza** (flu) and the common cold!

Coronaviruses are named for their crown of spikes. ("Corona" means "crown.") A kind of coronavirus also causes SARS, which stands for "severe acute respiratory syndrome," in humans. In late 2002, SARS spread from Asia through many parts of the world, causing **quarantines** and other safety measures. However, the outbreak was controlled by the end of July 2003. Fewer than 800 people died from SARS.

The illness was similar in some ways to COVID-19. Scientists believe that SARS started in a kind of bat or another animal and then jumped to humans. COVID-19 may have done the same.

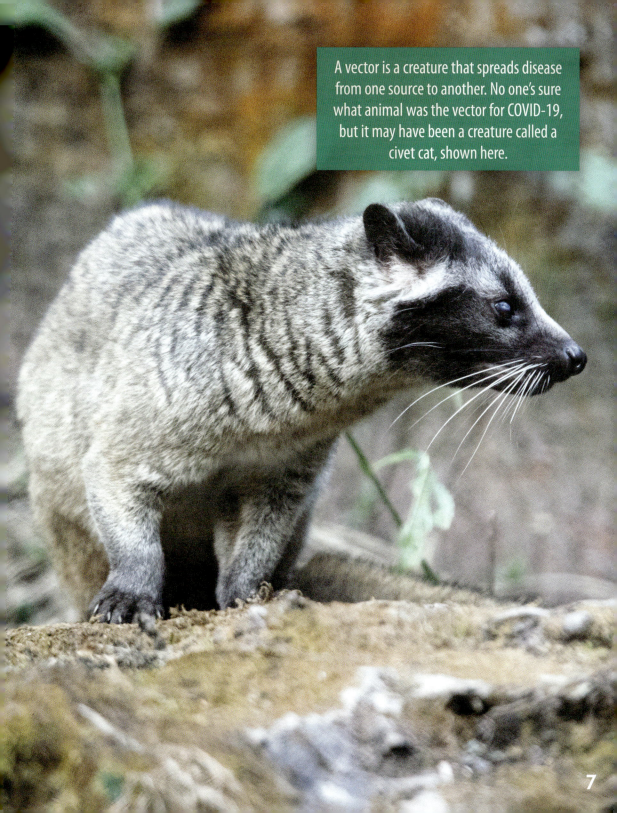

A vector is a creature that spreads disease from one source to another. No one's sure what animal was the vector for COVID-19, but it may have been a creature called a civet cat, shown here.

CHAPTER THREE

EPIDEMICS IN HISTORY

There have been many epidemics and pandemics throughout human history, including those caused by illnesses such as **cholera**, the flu, and **plague**. Perhaps the best-known plague is the Black Death, which hit Europe in the 14th century. It may have killed one-fourth to one-third of the population—as many as 25 million people. It was probably spread by fleas carried by rats.

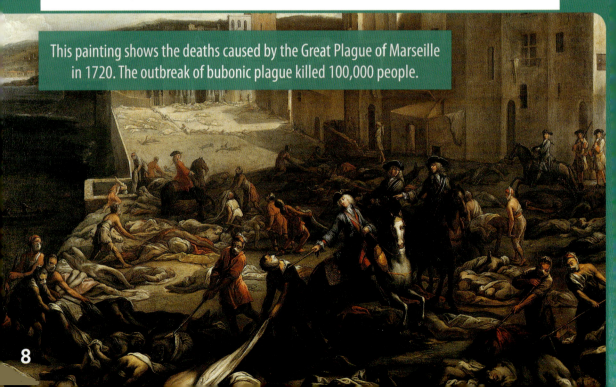

This painting shows the deaths caused by the Great Plague of Marseille in 1720. The outbreak of bubonic plague killed 100,000 people.

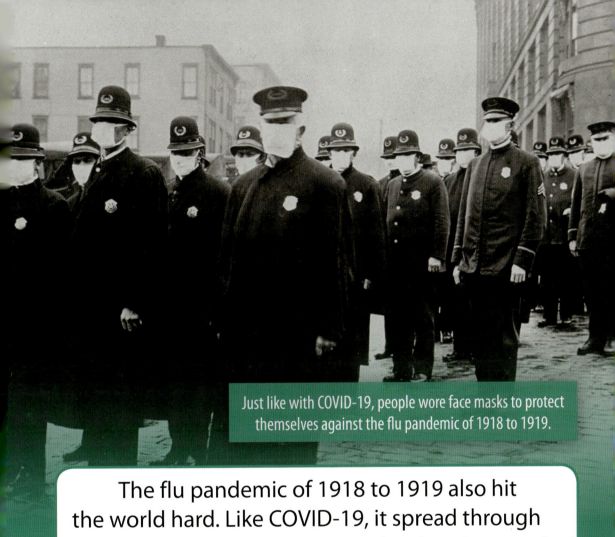

Just like with COVID-19, people wore face masks to protect themselves against the flu pandemic of 1918 to 1919.

The flu pandemic of 1918 to 1919 also hit the world hard. Like COVID-19, it spread through people by airborne respiratory droplets. It spread very quickly because World War I meant there were many soldiers close together. Millions of people—perhaps up to 100 million—died. Other epidemics—including AIDS, MERS (Middle East respiratory syndrome), and the Ebola virus—have happened since then. Still, few people seemed to expect the rise of COVID-19.

CHAPTER FOUR

LEARNING FROM THE PAST

For every sickness humanity has dealt with over the years, there have been lessons too. Over time, people learned more about the science behind health and illness. As time went on, the idea of public health—the art and science of protecting and improving community health through **sanitation**, preventative measures, and use of science—began to take shape. John Snow, a doctor in London during the mid-1800s, became known as "the father of **epidemiology**" for his work investigating the start and spread of cholera epidemics. He believed the disease was caused by germs instead of bad air, and he proved it with study.

More recent epidemics and pandemics have taught us lessons too. The 1918 flu pandemic showed scientists and historians that social distancing helped keep the sickness from spreading.

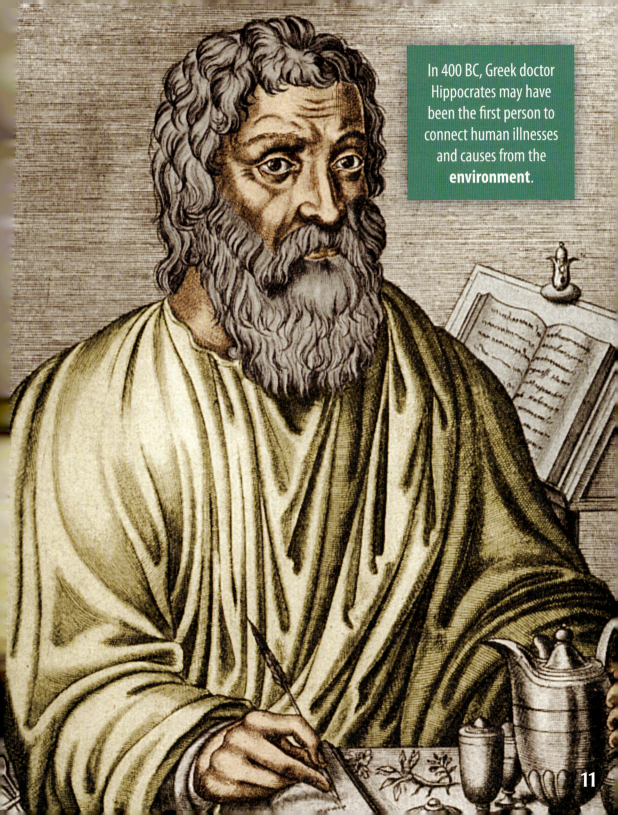

In 400 BC, Greek doctor Hippocrates may have been the first person to connect human illnesses and causes from the **environment**.

CHAPTER FIVE
COVID-19 APPEARS

Chinese officials reported the first cases of COVID-19 on December 31, 2019, but the sickness likely had been around longer than that. **Symptoms** were reported as fever, cough, and shortness of breath.

Epidemiologists looked for the cause. It turned out that many of the infected people had visited a live animal market in Wuhan, China. Scientists working with the samples discovered the sickness was caused by a new coronavirus.

COVID-19 (short for "coronavirus disease 2019") spread quickly. People began to die. Soon, China faced an epidemic. By mid-January, there were **confirmed** cases outside the country.

By January 23, Chinese officials ordered a lockdown in Wuhan and a few other cities. A week later, the World Health Organization (WHO) declared a "public health emergency of global concern" because of COVID-19.

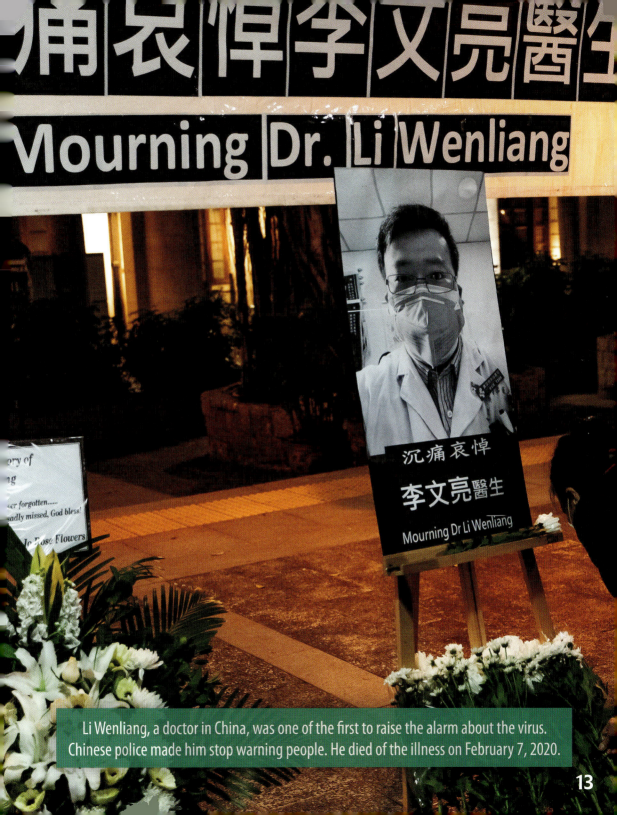

Li Wenliang, a doctor in China, was one of the first to raise the alarm about the virus. Chinese police made him stop warning people. He died of the illness on February 7, 2020.

CHAPTER SIX

THE VIRUS SPREADS

By the end of January, there were COVID-19 cases in many countries, including the United States. By February, people outside China started to die from the illness.

Scientists studied more about the illness and the virus. In time, scientists discovered that people could have COVID-19 for one to 14 days before they showed signs of it. That means people can spread the virus long before they know they have it. In fact, some people may be able to spread COVID-19 without any symptoms at all.

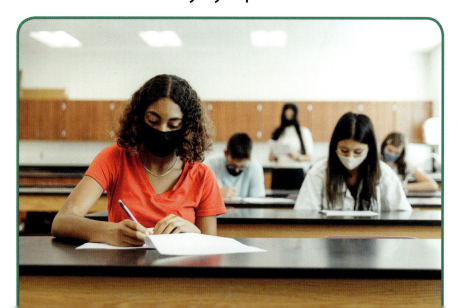

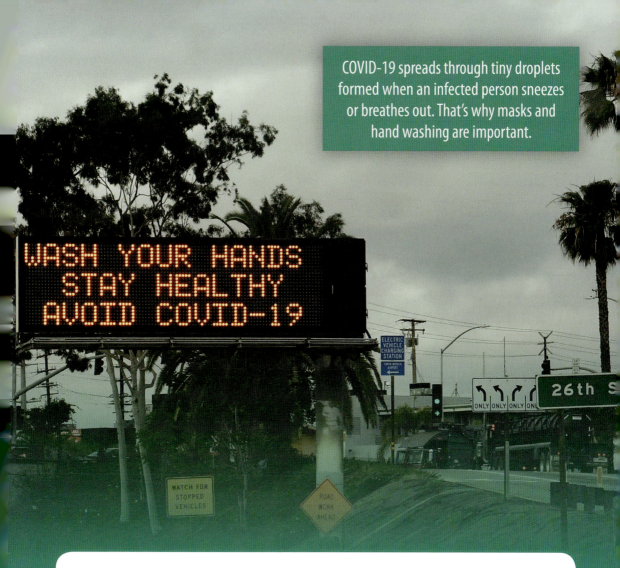

COVID-19 spreads through tiny droplets formed when an infected person sneezes or breathes out. That's why masks and hand washing are important.

On March 11, the World Health Organization announced that the COVID-19 outbreak was officially considered a pandemic. This was because of how fast the illness spread—and because of the inaction of some governments. At the time, there were more than 118,000 cases. More than 4,000 people had died.

CHAPTER SEVEN

WHAT HAPPENED IN ITALY

Although there were warnings, some world leaders and others didn't seem to realize just how dangerous COVID-19 could be. Italian officials closed down many events in the country by late February. However, the virus continued to spread, and soon, officials put a number of areas under a strict quarantine. Still, by the end of March, the death toll in Italy had passed 10,000.

There were a few reasons why the virus became such a problem there during this first wave. Many politicians didn't want to take action early on. Some people didn't listen to experts or follow quarantines at first. Officials also put safety measures in place little by little instead of all at once. That let the virus get started in the country and then spread.

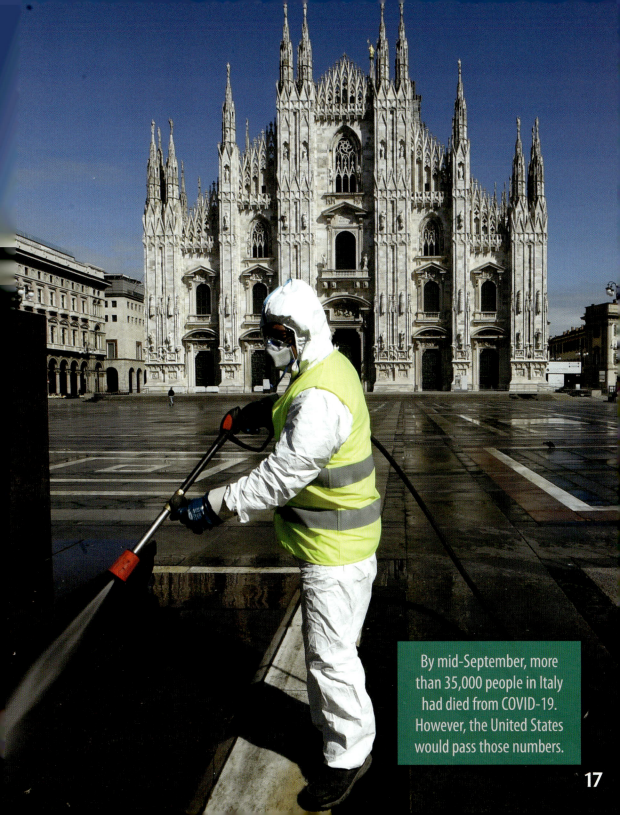

By mid-September, more than 35,000 people in Italy had died from COVID-19. However, the United States would pass those numbers.

17

CHAPTER EIGHT

COMING TO AMERICA

The first known case of COVID-19 in the United States was confirmed on January 21, 2020, in Washington State. The man had recently traveled to Wuhan, China. The first COVID-19 death in the United States occurred on February 6 in California.

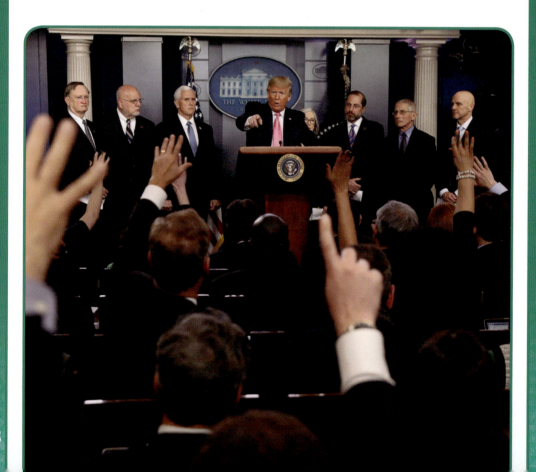

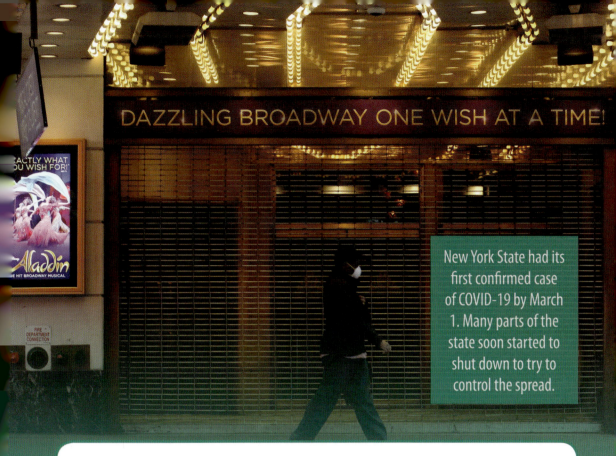

New York State had its first confirmed case of COVID-19 by March 1. Many parts of the state soon started to shut down to try to control the spread.

As in Italy, many U.S. officials and residents didn't think COVID-19 was much of a threat at first. However, the virus was already spreading across the country. There was a lot of confusion. Every state dealt with the outbreaks in different ways. Testing for the virus didn't work very well. Some states started to close schools to try to stop the spread.

By March 17, all 50 states had cases of the virus. There had been more than 100 known deaths and more than 6,000 cases.

CHAPTER NINE
COAST TO COAST

By March 20, New York was the center of the COVID-19 outbreak in the United States. Its conditions had become so bad, so fast, in part because the state and city shut down too late to control the rise. California, on the other hand, shut down when there were far fewer cases there. There may also have been other factors, such as population wealth, population **density**, and race. African Americans seem to be hit worse by COVID-19, and New York has a higher African American population.

However, cases in New York then slowed thanks to the shutdown. California, on the other hand, had issues once it started to reopen in May 2020. Many people began to act like the virus was gone, and it began to spread quickly again. Case numbers soon passed those in New York State.

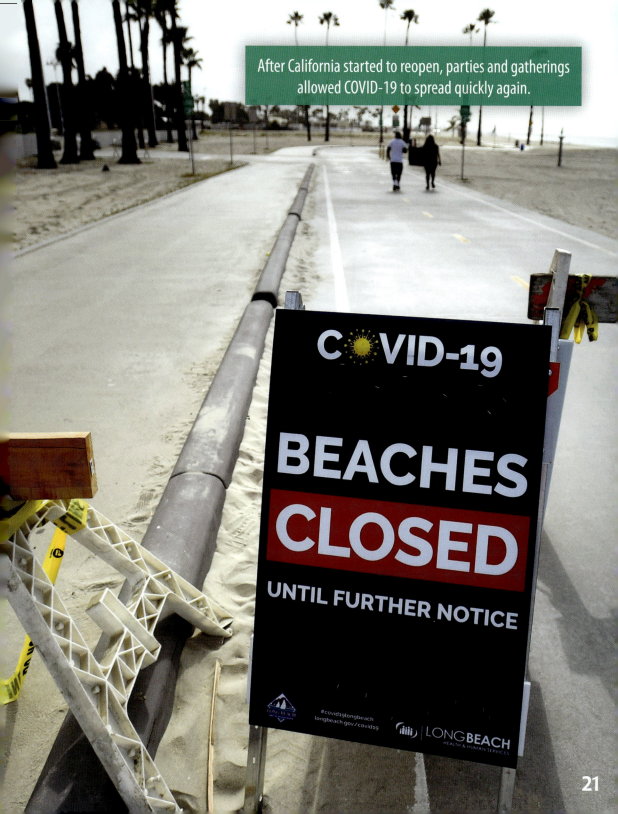
After California started to reopen, parties and gatherings allowed COVID-19 to spread quickly again.

CHAPTER TEN

TAKING SIDES

By March 26, 2020, the United States passed China to lead the world in COVID-19 cases. Some health organization directors say that the United States went wrong with its COVID-19 reaction in a few different ways. Many leaders denied COVID-19 was a threat. Some scientists noted a lack of government trust in science that could have helped the situation.

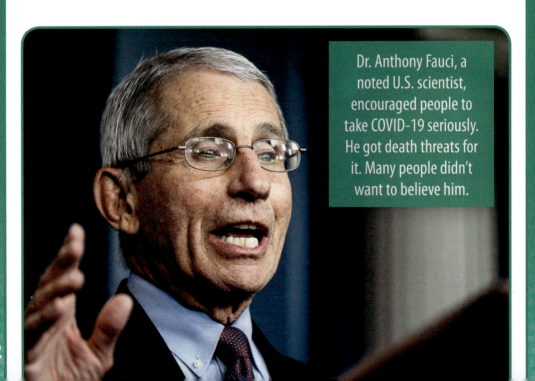

Dr. Anthony Fauci, a noted U.S. scientist, encouraged people to take COVID-19 seriously. He got death threats for it. Many people didn't want to believe him.

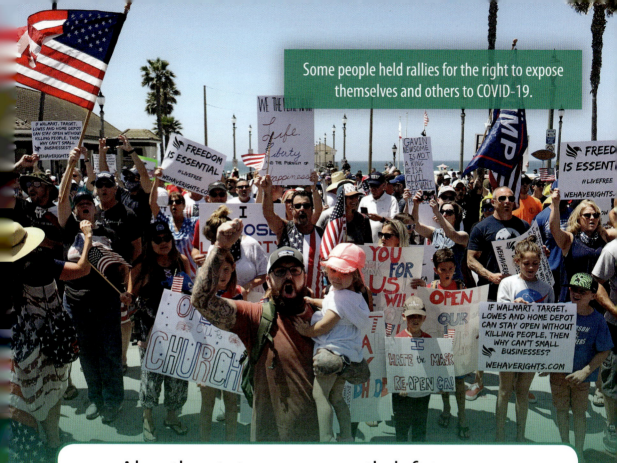

Some people held rallies for the right to expose themselves and others to COVID-19.

Also, the states were mostly left to themselves to figure out responses, testing, closures, and reopenings. Reopening too soon meant big increases in cases of the illness, although some politicians pushed for reopening to help the economy in an election year.

Some people rebelled against wearing face masks and social distancing. These measures can keep COVID-19 from spreading, but many politicians (including President Trump) suggested that they were against American freedoms.

CHAPTER ELEVEN
THE ISSUE OF MASKS

People are split widely on the issue of using face masks to prevent the spread of COVID-19. At first, many public health officials didn't say that people should wear masks. Especially early in the pandemic, many medical personnel had trouble getting good masks because of issues with the United States supply. Officials warned people against hoarding them because they were needed for health-care workers.

However, science-based **recommendations** can change as scientists learn more. They continued to study the way COVID-19 spread and learned that masks could help prevent the spread of the tiny, virus-laden particles that can infect people.

With this **information**, public health officials started saying that people should wear masks when around others. Some states and communities began to require masks when in public. However, some people still fought these rules.

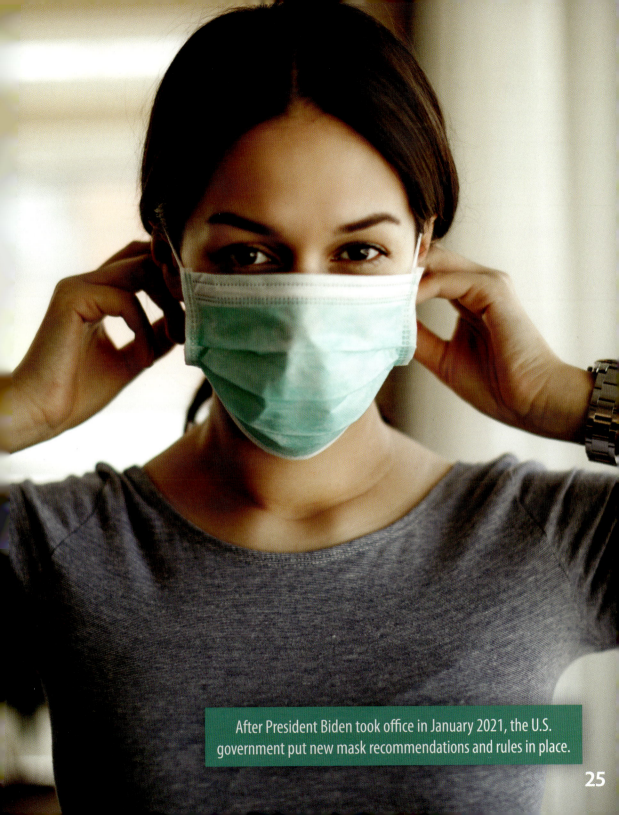

After President Biden took office in January 2021, the U.S. government put new mask recommendations and rules in place.

CHAPTER TWELVE

HOPE THROUGH SCIENCE

Many people who get COVID-19 probably won't have bad symptoms. Some people have no symptoms at all. However, some people will get very ill and need to stay in the hospital. Some die from the illness.

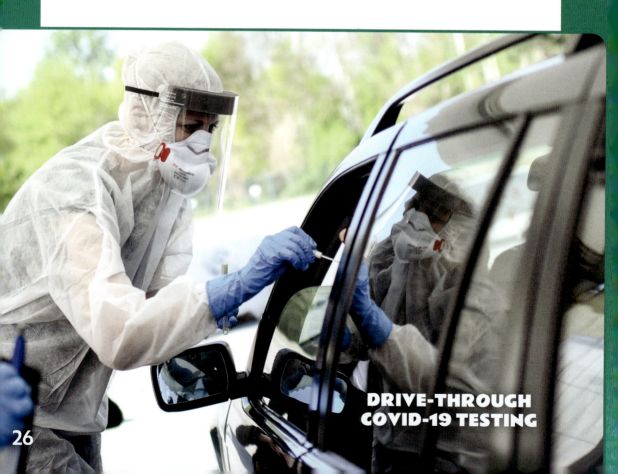

DRIVE-THROUGH COVID-19 TESTING

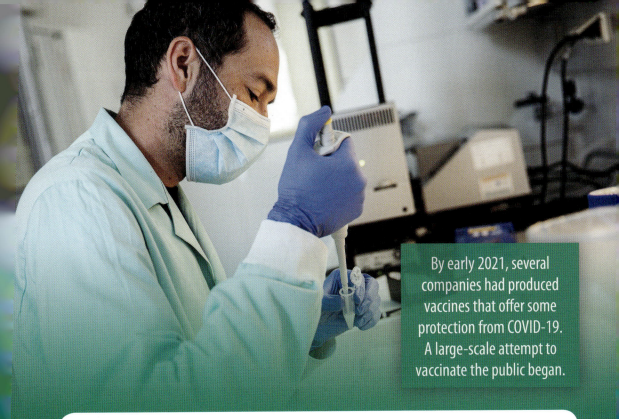

By early 2021, several companies had produced vaccines that offer some protection from COVID-19. A large-scale attempt to vaccinate the public began.

Doctors also still aren't sure what the full aftereffects of COVID-19 might be. The virus can damage the heart, lungs, and brain, although scientists are still studying the long-term effects.

There was a great deal of hope in the beginning of 2021, however. A few companies have produced vaccines that seem to work well against COVID-19. By early 2021, efforts to vaccinate the U.S. population were underway. Also, in late October 2020, the U.S. Food and Drug Administration (FDA) approved the first drug, remdesivir, to be used in treating COVID-19.

CHAPTER THIRTEEN
LOOK FOR THE HELPERS

The COVID-19 pandemic has been hard, but many young people have stepped up to make a difference. Avi Schiffmann, a teenager from Washington State, created a COVID-19 tracker online (ncov2019.live/data), one so thorough that scientists have used it. He had help from a team of other teenagers from around the world. Some young journalists joined the Teenage Reporting Project COVID-19 (www.globalyouthandnewsmediaprize.net/project-world-teenage-reporting-pro). The project has included many stories about young people doing their best to make a difference in many ways.

Some young people have found new ways to create protective equipment to help in the COVID-19 fight. Claire Kang of the United States was one of the teenagers who started Washington Youth for Masks to provide safety equipment to hospitals. Other students have created face masks with 3-D printers.

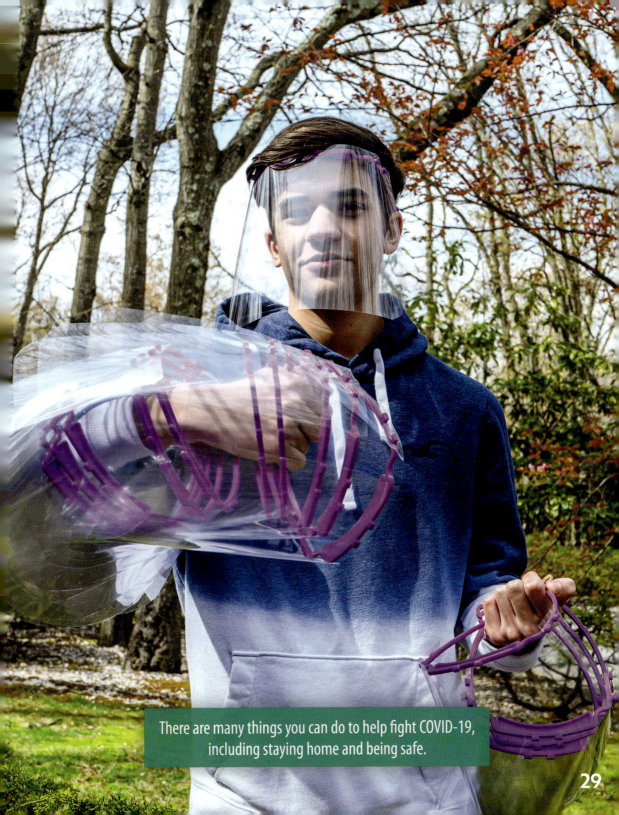

There are many things you can do to help fight COVID-19, including staying home and being safe.

29

CHAPTER FOURTEEN

INTO THE FUTURE

With the rise of COVID-19, the world changed forever. As of late February 2021, there have been more than 26 million cases in the United States, and more than 500,000 people have died. Worldwide, there have been more than 106 million cases and more than 2.3 million deaths. The United States continues to have the highest number of cases and deaths in the world.

Things are different for everyone, including young people. No one truly knows just what the future will look like. However, new United States leaders, including President Biden, have already outlined new plans for fighting the pandemic. Vaccines have been developed, and many people have already been vaccinated. There is hope.

Together, we can make it through this pandemic and into a post-COVID-19 future.

GLOSSARY

cholera (KAH-luh-ruh) A deadly disease often caused by a bacterium and marked by stomach and intestinal problems.

confirm (kuhn-FUHRM) To state or show that something is correct.

density (DEHN-suh-tee) The amount of a something in a given area, such as people in a town or country.

environment (ihn-VY-ruhn-munht) The natural world around us.

epidemiology (eh-puh-dee-mee-AH-luh-jee) A branch of medical science that deals with disease in a population.

influenza (in-flu-EHN-zuh) A sickness that can include fever, upset stomach, and aches and pains; also known as the flu.

information (in-fuhr-MAY-shuhn) Knowledge or facts about something.

particle (PAAR-tih-kuhl) One of the very small parts of matter.

plague (PLAYG) A disease that spreads from person to person quickly and kills many people.

quarantine (KWOHR-uhn-teen) Keeping something away from the public to stop the spread of disease. Also, to keep something away from the public to stop the spread of disease.

recommendation (reh-kuh-muhn-DAY-shuhn) A suggestion about what should be done.

sanitation (sa-nuh-TAY-shuhn) The process of keeping places free from dirt and disease.

symptom (SIMP-tuhm) A sign that shows someone is sick.

INDEX

A
AIDS, 9

B
Biden, Joseph, 25, 30

C
California, 18, 20, 21
China, 4, 12, 13, 14, 18, 22
cholera, 8, 10

E
Ebola virus, 9
epidemiology, 10

F
Fauci, Anthony, 22
Food and Drug Administration (FDA), 27

H
Hippocrates, 11

I
influenza (flu), 6, 8, 9, 10
Italy, 16, 19

K
Kang, Claire, 28

L
Li Wenliang, 13

M
MERS, 9

N
New York State, 19, 20

P
plague, 8

S
SARS, 6
Schiffmann, Avi, 28
Snow, John, 10

T
Trump, Donald, 23

U
United States, 14, 17, 18, 19, 20, 22, 24, 28, 30

V
vaccines, 27, 30

W
Washington State, 18, 28
World Health Organization (WHO), 12, 15
World War I, 9
Wuhan, 6, 12, 18

PRIMARY SOURCE LIST

Page 9
Policemen wearing face masks during the flu epidemic. Photograph. 1918. Seattle, Washington. Held by Time Life Pictures.

Page 11
Portrait of Hippocrates. Painting. ca. 400 BC. Held by Getty Images.

Page 29
Brandon Gregory and face masks he created. Photograph. 2020. Dix Hills, New York. Alejandra Villa Loarca. Held by Getty Images.

WEBSITES

Due to the changing nature of Internet links, PowerKids Press has developed an online list of websites related to the subject of this book. This site is updated regularly. Please use this link to access the list: www.powerkidslinks.com/SOOF/pandemic